ENDOMETRIUM

*My Journey Through
Endometrial Cancer*

OLIVIA TUSK

ISBN: 978-1-7385822-9-7

TABLE OF CONTENTS

1 - The Symptoms

2 - The Ultrasound

3 - The Pipelle Biopsy

4 - The Confirmation

5 - The MRI

6 - The Discussions

7 - The Laporascopic Hysterectomy

8 - Surgical Follow Up

9 - Wound Issues

10 - Counselling Session

11 - The Bleeding

12 - The Pre-Radiation Checkup

13 - The Radiation

14 - Post Radiation

15 - Follow Up

1
The Symptoms

Thursday, July 28th, 2022. That was the evening that I noticed a discharge that wasn't like one I'd had before. Even though I'd last had a menstrual period four years earlier, so was considered as being in full menopause, discharges were still fairly common. I'd grown used to these and generally thought nothing of them, but seeing this one have a slight bloody tinge to it - not a full-on bleed, but enough of that coloration to make me look closer at it - made me curious.

Onto the Internet I went. While I try to keep an open mind about anything I read online, when I'd seen enough websites suggesting that anything resembling a bleed after being in menopause was worth seeing a GP about, I took heed. First thing Monday, I called to make an appointment. Tuesday, I was in my doctor's office, being reassured that I'd done the right thing to go in and chat to her about it.

In and around the interim of this little bleed - and it was only a very little bleed, with that one small amount of spotting being the ONLY sign that my body gave me to say something was wrong - I investigated more about the possible causes of such an event to take place.

Endometrial Cancer. The words kept leaping out at me while I was researching online, but it was a cancer I'd never heard of. Since being told at the age of sixteen that my mother had been diagnosed with breast cancer, I'd always had a wariness about 'the big C' throughout my life to date. For that whole time, from age sixteen till my diagnosis age of 52, I thought I'd done everything right as far as cancer went. I'd had breast checks since my mid-twenties - ultrasounds at first, and then mammograms, almost yearly. I'd gotten smear tests done annually, instead of the recommended frequency. I honestly thought that by being so proactive in getting these kinds of tests done, I might be able to stop cancer in its path, even if I couldn't stop it from trying to get me. But this particular kind of cancer, I'd never even heard of. Imagine my surprise, then, when I was doing my online research and found out that endometrial cancer is one of the most common cancers in women. What? I'd been seeing ads on TV for years about getting this checked or that checked, for several kinds of cancer, but there hadn't been any mention at all about this one, and it was common? It seemed silly, to say the least. I mean, if you're going to look right up inside me to do a smear test, you couldn't just do another scraping of my uterus lining while in the general vicinity? No, it wasn't that simple apparently, even though it seemed that obvious in my flawed logic.

Talking to my GP, she was really good at helping me gain a better understanding of what might be happening inside of me. She explained that bleeding after menopause *could* be a symptom of this cancer, but not to get too ahead of myself and worry too much. That was a difficult thing to do. I'd been sixteen when I'd first learned about cancer at all, with my mother being diagnosed with her breast cancer. I'd been eighteen when she'd died. I'd been just that right age to have the equation cemented into my head:

Cancer = death

Now, taking a step back and forcing myself to look at statistics and general medical reports, I could see that lots of people get cancer and survive. My child mind wanted to argue with that logic simply because that equation had been sitting in the back of my memory for decades. I can easily admit just how difficult it was for me to even consider the possibility that I might survive if I was diagnosed with cancer.

But the first part was dealt with. I'd had some faint blood in a discharge on one evening, and my GP was going to recommend I go and get an ultrasound done of my pelvic region, specifically to do a measurement of my uterus lining. How that could tell anyone anything, I had no idea, but a couple of days later, I received my appointment date.

Your notes:

If you think it might be helpful in any way, either now or in the future, use this space to record your own experience and feelings at this point.

……………………………………………………...

……………………………………………………...

……………………………………………………...

……………………………………………………...

……………………………………………………...

……………………………………………………...

……………………………………………………...

……………………………………………………...

……………………………………………………...

……………………………………………………...

……………………………………………………...

2
The Ultrasound

Monday, August 8th, 2022. To say that I was relieved to get an appointment so quickly for the ultrasound to be done is an understatement. For almost a week I'd been worrying and, by then, I have to say, I'd actually begun to think about what to do if I got the diagnosis. What would I prioritize to make the most of whatever time I had left? I was getting too ahead of myself, but that thought had already begun to settle on my mind. It took a lot to tell myself that I might have cancer, and I might go on to die from it, but I wasn't likely to die from it *that day*. Generally, I felt perfectly fine, and perfectly normal. If my body hadn't shown me that one small moment of bloody discharge, I really wouldn't have known anything was wrong at all.

     The ultrasound was easy and painless, as they most often are. It was a quick appointment, in and out, with reassurance from the staff that I'd know of their findings within a short period of time.

With a brief trip already planned for the following week to head away and do a fun run, I went off and did that, and continued to feel fine. Nothing about any other aspect of my health and body told me something was going on inside of me that wasn't great.

When my GP let me know that the ultrasound had shown some thickening in my uterus wall, she also told me she was putting through a referral for me to get a Pipelle biopsy. Again, it was something I'd never heard of, but I understood it had to be done.

This was where the waiting period begun. For two months, my GP maintained contact with me, asking each week if I'd received an appointment from the clinic she'd referred me to. Every time I told her I hadn't, she was wonderfully proactive in chasing them up. When two months had passed, she decided to put my case into the public hospital system instead of waiting for the smaller clinic to do the biopsy. Once I was in the public hospital system, things started to move along once again.

Your notes:

If you think it might be helpful in any way, either now or in the future, use this space to record your own experience and feelings at this point.

. . . .

. . . .

. . . .

. . . .

. . . .

. . . .

. . . .

. . . .

. . . .

. . . .

. . . .

3
The Pipelle Biopsy

Wednesday, November 2nd, 2022. When I got my appointment for this biopsy, I didn't think much of it. Sitting down with the gynecology surgeon who was going to do it, she was wonderful in explaining what she was going to do. To me, it sounded just like any other smear test. I was pretty surprised by the ways it *wasn't* just like a smear test, but as with any kind of test 'down there', it was just a matter of having to breathe deeply and get through it.

I won't lie - the biopsy procedure wasn't pleasant. Being in the position of feet up in stirrups, and being open for all to see, is something that tests the dignity of all of us. That side of things isn't nice, but it's acceptable to me for living in a time when we are fortunate to have pretty incredible health care available to us. In truth, it was the discomfort that was the surprise. In smear tests, I've always found that I can feel that little scraping of the cervix when it's done. In this biopsy, it was like that, but of a much bigger degree. For almost half an hour, it felt like it went on and on, but as horrible as I found it, I just had to keep telling myself that it'd be over with soon enough and once it was, that would be the end of that particular chore - it wouldn't have to be done again.

Thirty minutes later, I was sat down as the gynecology surgeon explained what could happen if things were as they thought it would be. It all sounded worrisome, but I did appreciate how straightforward she was in speaking to me and making sure I understood that I was the one in charge of decisions that might lay ahead. With many kinds of cancer, everyone is entitled to have treatment, but not everyone wants it. While she informed me that the results weren't yet known for sure, she was fairly confident that my uterus lining could contain some cancer, but she was also confident that if that was the case, it was entirely curable. I walked away from that appointment hopeful. Whatever the diagnosis, maybe it wouldn't be a death sentence.

Over the two days following the Pipelle biopsy, I experienced a lot of bleeding, but this had been explained as perfectly normal and to be expected. While it was weird having what seemed like a period, after so long of not having had to worry about such things, I had to keep thinking ahead. I'm a mum. I might be leaving my son earlier rather than later, depending on how things would go, but then again, I might not. It was a timely reminder that, no matter how long I had to live, I had been remiss in setting up lots of things and putting them in place for when I leave this world. Maybe it isn't be a bad thing to have little reminders like this. Our time is coming for all of us. It's easy to get so caught up in living today that we overlook making things easy for our kids when our time comes. Needless to say, while waiting for results from the biopsy, it turned out to be a great time to get on and get a few things in order that should have already been done years earlier.

Your notes:

If you think it might be helpful in any way, either now or in the future, use this space to record your own experience and feelings at this point.

....

....

....

....

....

....

....

....

....

....

4
The Confirmation

Monday, November 14th, 2022. The call from the surgeon came on an afternoon when I was at a friend's house. There's something powerful about hearing the words, 'are you sitting down?'. When I heard them, I knew it was going to be a positive result for the endometrial cancer. The surgeon was good to talk to, explaining that she recommended I go in to have a laparoscopic hysterectomy, and that once it was done, the cancer would be gone and that would be that.

Despite there being options for other forms of treatment, I was happy to go and have a full hysterectomy. My periods were over with and my baby making days had been over for years, so it wasn't a difficult choice at all. Although the surgeon kept saying that after it was all cut out, I would be cancer free, my child mind kept all the concern alive in me. Sure, they might be removing my uterus altogether, and therefore cutting out the cancer they'd found there, but cancer could be anywhere else in my body, for all I knew. If my body hadn't released one tiny spot of blood, or if I hadn't noticed it, I would have been continuing through life, not knowing my uterus was slowly succumbing to the cells turning cancerous. Who was to say that my entire body wasn't riddled with the stuff if no signs were given.

News delivered and knowledge of surgery option explained, it was just another waiting period. Fortunately, I live in a country where medical attention through the public hospital system is timely and fairly fast, especially considering how many people need to be in hospital on any given day.

Before surgery could take place, only two more things needed to be done - an MRI of my entire pelvic area, and an x-ray of my chest and upper torso. Both sounded easy enough. I was eager to get on with it, and get it all over with.

Your notes:

If you think it might be helpful in any way, either now or in the future, use this space to record your own experience and feelings at this point.

…………………………………………………..

…………………………………………………..

…………………………………………………..

…………………………………………………..

…………………………………………………..

…………………………………………………..

…………………………………………………..

…………………………………………………..

…………………………………………………..

…………………………………………………..

…………………………………………………...

5
The MRI

Tuesday, November 29th, 2022. Walking into the hospital radiology department to get ready for a chest x-ray and an MRI of my pelvis wasn't scary at all. I'd never had either, but knew people who had. Nobody had ever said either hurt, so I wasn't concerned.

When it came time to have the MRI done, everything sounded fine. Even as the two medical staff members prepared me for going into the machine, I felt relaxed. I continued to feel relaxed until I was fully inside of it. Even though it was open at either end, and there was plenty of air, and I was safe with nothing happening to me, within a couple of minutes I was screaming for them to pull me out.

It was a weird experience, but the ladies were wonderful, giving me time to get my breathing under control and ready myself to try again. The second time I attempted it, I made sure to keep my eyes closed. I felt the slat I was on move, and I could hear the staff talking to me through the headphones they'd provided, along with some dubious music choices. It took effort to not open my eyes in case doing so put me into a panic attack again. For the most part, all it took for my effort was to lie still. That, combined with a few episodes of having to hold my breath for what felt like far too long, was all it took. The noises the machine made were horrid, but I knew I had to persist. The more still I could be, the sooner I'd be out of there and hopefully wouldn't have to ever go back in. That was enough for me to commit to doing just that.

When they pulled me out of the machine, I breathed easily again, with the resolve that I really didn't like having an MRI taken. It is not in any way cool at all! But at least it was done. Quarter of an hour later, the chest x-ray was taken as well (far less stressful), and then I walked out into the sunshine. As horrible as the experience was, I felt blessed that things continued to be moving along at a good pace.

Your notes:

*If you think it might be helpful in any way,
either now or in the future, use this space to
record your own experience and
feelings at this point.*

....

....

....

....

....

....

....

....

....

....

....

6
The Discussions

Tuesday, December 1st, 2022. The first discussion I had to have, before surgery would be finalized, was with the anaestheologist. Many questions were asked during this appointment but, overall, it was a simple thing to get through. Fifteen minutes was all it took for them to get from me all they needed, and for me to know what I needed to do in the 24 hours leading up to surgery.

On Monday, 5 December 2022, I met with the gynecology surgeon again. Although I'd already said that I was happy to go through with the full hysterectomy, it was nice to be sat down and asked again if I was sure. No matter what other options might have been out there for other people to explore in the same situation, I knew that I was happy with the surgery option. Although the surgeon was confident that the cancer was in the first 50% of the uterus lining, so the hysterectomy would effectively 'cure' me of cancer, she did also explain that they wouldn't be entirely certain until they got in there and could examine the uterus further. The news didn't upset me. I was already in a state of 'might survive this, or might not' kind of thinking.

Your notes:

If you think it might be helpful in any way, either now or in the future, use this space to record your own experience and feelings at this point.

....

....

....

....

....

....

....

....

....

....

....

7
The Laporascopic Hysterectomy

Monday, December 12th, 2022. Being admitted into hospital is something I've never done in my lifetime, except to give birth to my son via caesarean. I wasn't sure exactly what to expect, but just like most aspects of my cancer journey, everything happened quite quickly. After being shown to a room to get changed into one of those attractive gowns, I was transported on a bed down to the operation theatre. There I waited for some time, with various medical staff coming to talk to me and then get me set up and ready for anaesthetic.

Once the surgeon had come and said hello, I was instructed to lie back as staff moved around me. After the mask was placed over my face, I drifted off.

I can still remember the moments of waking up after the surgery was complete. Hazy moments of people talking to me, saying it was time to wake up, eventually evened out into wakefulness. At first I couldn't understand what was happening. I'd gone into surgery just after 12pm. The time on the clock in front of me when I was fully awake said 6.30pm. I'd thought the surgery would only be a couple of hours.

After fully waking and being checked over, I was moved to a ward. In the hospital, I stayed for two nights/one day. During that time, I felt like everything was perfectly normal, and like there wasn't going to be any pain at all. Of course, once I got home, I realized I hadn't felt any pain during my time in hospital because they'd kept giving me so many painkillers. Settled in back at home again, the pain was felt pretty quickly!

Following my hospital stay, I was instructed to take things very easy and let my body begin to recover. No lifting, no straining, and generally not doing very much at all. They were the instructions I was given, and I gave it a good go to try and follow them. It was difficult since I felt some pain, but Paracetamol proved sufficient for my meager pain needs. It was mostly difficult to not do anything, even though that always sounds good in theory.

Your notes:

If you think it might be helpful in any way, either now or in the future, use this space to record your own experience and feelings at this point.

....

....

....

....

....

....

....

....

....

....

....

8
Surgical Follow Up

Friday, December 23rd, 2022. Meeting with a member of the gynaecology surgery team, I was informed that while they'd expected the cancer to have been caught in the first 50% of my uterus lining, once they'd removed the uterus and fully tested it, they'd found it was instead exactly *at* 50%. When they said that, all I kept thinking was that if my body hadn't given me that one small sign that something was going on, how quickly would the cancer have continued to move through the rest of the lining and into other nearby parts of my body? It made me further grateful that my body did alert me to something needing to be checked, and that I did sit up and take notice.

With the health system in my country, the guideline for whether radiation would be advised following the hysterectomy or not, is whether the cancer has been caught within the first 50% of the lining or not. In my case, with it sitting exactly at 50%, it was decided to treat that as over 50%. It was recommended to me that I complete some radiation treatment of the top of the vagina. Nothing had been found there. It was purely a 'just in case' option.

I won't lie. Being given a 'just in case' option for radiation wasn't an easy choice. Yes, if there were some little cancer cells still lurking around that area, the radiation would deal to them. On the other hand, it was explained to me that radiation can also *cause* cancer. I could end up getting cancer in a location where there wasn't any, purely from the treatment. It wasn't an easy decision to make, but I decided to follow their suggestion and get it done. It was also recommended to me that I take advantage of the three sessions of counselling that the hospital could offer as part of cancer support. I didn't think I'd need that, but again decided to follow their guidelines.

While talking to the member of the gynaecology surgery team, I had to ask quite a few questions. For most of my life, I'd been getting smear tests to check for cancer in there. After surgery, I no longer *have* any bits to check each year. How would I know if there was cancer in there from that point forward? It was reassuring to hear that I'd be getting six monthly checkups pretty much for the rest of my life through the hospital system. To quote the words of the medical staff member who spoke to me: "you're stuck with us now!".

Your notes:

If you think it might be helpful in any way, either now or in the future, use this space to record your own experience and feelings at this point.

....

....

....

....

....

....

....

....

....

....

9
Wound Issues

Tuesday, January 17th, 2023. In the weeks after my gynaecology surgery check up, I started to notice one of my four wounds (the four laporascopic wounds being two on either side of my navel, one in the naval itself, and one under my belly) was painful and looked like it might be infected. A quick visit to the hospital resulted in the wound being swabbed, and later showing a staph infection. Great.

　　When I was able to get in to see my GP and have the wound checked again, I was put onto a course of antibiotics to deal with that. It was painful for a few more days, but slowly I could see it was starting to mend itself. Again, it was a period of being told to rest and not lift anything or do much, to prevent the wound being pulled apart. Once again, it was hard to do nothing, but obviously I'd done more than I should have once I'd come home from the hospital after surgery. I was determined to sit still for however many days it would take for the wound to heal properly.

Your notes:

If you think it might be helpful in any way, either now or in the future, use this space to record your own experience and feelings at this point.

....

....

....

....

....

....

....

....

....

....

....

10
Counselling Session

Wednesday, January 18th, 2023. Talking to counsellors is something I've never indulged in, so it was difficult to know what exactly to talk to one about.

The woman assigned to me was lovely, prompting me to speak about how I was feeling about the cancer, and about how things were going in my home because of it. It definitely opened up some interesting thought pathways, and although I didn't ask to use another of the three sessions that had been made available to me, it was a worthwhile activity.

I'd recommend to anyone in this situation to take advantage of at least the first counselling session that's offered. It can feel nice to have a total stranger for a sounding board, instead of feeling like talking to friends or family would only weigh them down.

Your notes:

If you think it might be helpful in any way, either now or in the future, use this space to record your own experience and feelings at this point.

....

....

....

....

....

....

....

....

....

....

....

11
The Bleeding

Thursday, January 19th, 2023. Five weeks after my hysterectomy, when things had started to feel a little bit normal again, I experienced an intense bleed. It wasn't slow, like a period. Although I didn't feel it happening at the time, I knew that it was over only a very short time that an extreme amount of blood had oozed out of me. Thankfully, my GP was at her computer doing paperwork when I sent a message to her via a health app, just letting her know that I'd had a big bleed.

When I sent the message, it was just to let her know, and I intended at that time to see the night out and just monitor if it was going to be an ongoing problem, or just one big gush that was already done with.

When I received a message back from her, I was surprised by the urgency of her words that instructed me to get to the hospital emergency department as soon as I could, and that she'd send through a letter to them to make sure I was prioritized when I got there. If I hadn't been worried about the bleed when it happened, I certainly was after hearing back from my GP. In her opinion, having a major bleed five weeks after a hysterectomy wasn't normal or anything to be ignored.

Following her instruction, I went to the hospital, where several staff members checked me out, and eventually decided to admit me for the night, just in case it was something serious. There I stayed overnight, and got to be examined by the original hysterectomy surgeon the following morning. Her response was that five weeks after a hysterectomy, it was perfectly *normal* to have a major bleed. This was in stark contrast to my GP's concern. But it was done, and at least I'd had the bleed checked and my mind put at rest again, even if I probably would have been fine at home for the night after all.

After the checkup was completed by the surgeon, I was allowed to return home. I felt tired from the blood loss and the night in the hospital but, as always, it was good to get home.

Your notes:

If you think it might be helpful in any way, either now or in the future, use this space to record your own experience and feelings at this point.

....

....

....

....

....

....

....

....

....

....

12
The Pre-Radiation Check-up

Monday, February 13th, 2023. After having travel and accommodation organized by my local public hospital, I ended up having to travel to another city and hospital to get radiation treatment. The equipment for this particular kind of radiation delivery - vaginal - isn't in my local hospital. With the health board taking full control of organizing everything, it was easy to travel and settle in for a week away.

The plan was for me to have a pre-radiation checkup on the Monday, and then have radiation given to me on the Tuesday, Thursday and Friday. That was the plan. That wasn't what ended up happening.

Before my dates of radiation had been finalized, the 'away' hospital had been informed about the bleed I'd had a few weeks earlier. They'd decided the cause of the bleeding - most likely, some vaginal stitches coming loose - would be fine and healed by the time my radiation treatment dates arrived.

When I arrived at the hospital for the pre-radiation checkup, I was put through a CT scan first, and then measurement of my vagina (yes, you read that right). As far as I understand, this is needed to make sure that the equipment the radiation is delivered through inside the vagina is the best possible fit - neither too tight nor too loose. It is a strange thing, being told the 'size' of your vagina, but as with every part of this journey, it was just a matter of nodding and smiling, and looking forward to the next step.

All was well until the radiation specialist did an internal exam. That was all it took to set off a new round of bleeding. After an hour or so of back and forth conversation between the gynaecology surgery department and the oncology department, it was decided to put off the radiation for a further ten days. It would mean a paid-for holiday in the city I was in, since there were no seats on any earlier flights to get me home, and then a return to the away-city the following week.

Since I have friends in that city, I didn't mind in the least that I was able to stay there all week in paid accommodation. It was this week that I also made the decision to begin to work towards building fitness again. I hadn't done anything physical since before the surgery - almost three months. During that week away, I started over again with a meager five rounds of 30 seconds walking and 30 seconds jogging. It was a tiny amount of movement, but it was the start of getting my body moving again. During that first week, I did a few little jog/walks like this. I've never truly been into fitness, but it really did feel good to be out in the fresh air in a park, and moving my body, even for so little amount of time.

Your notes:

If you think it might be helpful in any way, either now or in the future, use this space to record your own experience and feelings at this point.

....

....

....

....

....

....

....

....

....

....

13
The Radiation

Friday, February 24th, 2023. After a week away, then less than a week at home, I travelled a second time to again try to get radiation done. This time, everything was fine.

During the first session, it was strange to be opened up and exposed to several people who were in the room with me, working together to get all of my body in the right position, and also get the equipment ready. On that first day, I just had to focus on breathing deeply and keeping calm. The equipment looked large, but relaxing helped to let the radiation staff insert it into the vagina.

Once the equipment was in place and the staff had all left the room, all that was required from me was to lie still and relax. It seemed to take maybe ten minutes (three songs on the radio). During that time, I could hear the innards of the equipment moving, I'm guessing to move as it delivered radiation outwards to the walls/top of the vagina. It wasn't painful at all, but it felt good when the staff returned and removed it. That was one day's radiation session. Very short, even if not very sweet.

After a weekend off, the process was repeated on Monday, February 27th, 2023, and Tuesday, February 28th, 2023. On none of these three sessions was there any difficulty. Before leaving, I was given a vaginal dilator and instructions on how to use that (and the importance of using it) after four weeks, and I was told the staff would ring me in four weeks to check how things were going.

Overall, the radiation treatment was fine in the delivery, and while I did feel a bit more tired than usual in the week afterward, it wasn't extreme.

Your notes:

*If you think it might be helpful in any way,
either now or in the future, use this space to
record your own experience and
feelings at this point.*

....

....

....

....

....

....

....

....

....

....

....

14
Post Radiation

The Dilator. After a couple of weeks had passed following the radiation treatment, it was time for me to begin to use the vaginal dilator I'd been given. It was a daunting task, even though it was nothing to worry about. All the dilator was is a set of plastic tubes of four different sizes, designed to be used to help keep the vagina open.

If I've understood correctly (forgive me if I haven't), after radiation and the trauma that's caused by it internally (kind of like getting sunburnt on the inside), the body can try to close up the walls of the vagina as a way of mending itself. The dilators are designed to be used to help to keep the vagina open and the walls apart.

I've never been one to self-insert hard plastic inside me, so I found it very odd to do this exercise, but I forced myself to. Starting with the skinniest tube, I did that for a few times, then graduated to the next size up, and then up to the third size. Being in a relationship, I opted to welcome back my partner to intimacy after that, with the fourth size of dilator looking just a little *too* big for my liking. Being sexual from that point onwards was no problem at all, and I'm sure that was partly because of having used the smaller dilators when I did. It's difficult to imagine the vagina mending itself from trauma by sealing itself up, but visualizing that was enough to inspire me to follow the guidelines for using the dilator, and then becoming sexual again.

Other than having to go through the process of keeping my vagina healthy, and a little bit of feeling the healing processing happening (similar to feeling a burn begin to heal) there were no other issues after radiation for me.

Your notes:

If you think it might be helpful in any way, either now or in the future, use this space to record your own experience and feelings at this point.

....

....

....

....

....

....

....

....

....

....

....

15
Follow Up

Monday, April 24th 2023. About seven weeks after the radiation treatment, I had my first check up with the hospital. This entailed a general question session, asking if I'd had any issues at all. After that, I was given the vaginal version of a smear test. I believe this will be what each six-monthly check up will entail from this point forward.

Your notes:

If you think it might be helpful in any way, either now or in the future, use this space to record your own experience and feelings at this point.

....

....

....

....

....

....

....

....

....

....

16
End Note

Through every stage of my journey, from that first tiny speck of blood in that discharge, right through to this follow up, I've met some wonderful people in various sections of the medical health service. Throughout my time in two hospitals, and with my GP, I've felt blessed to live in a country where medical care is free to the general public, and so attentive in getting me through the system as quickly as I was.

So why have I written this short outline of my experience? Only so that maybe you are on a journey like me, and wonder what might lay ahead. Even if you are, your journey may not be the same as mine. What you have to go through might not be the same as what I did, or you might not live somewhere that can provide as quick health care as what I've received.

What I'd like to come most of all from my journey, is people simply knowing about this cancer. I knew nothing - I'd never even heard of it. I feel blessed that my body gave me a sign, even if it was only one and it was tiny. I want other people to know about this cancer, and to learn the symptoms and signs of it.

If you're a woman, or you're a man with special women in your life, I hope you'll take a moment to go online and do some reading. If you experience - or if you hear of another woman talking about the same kind of experience - of a small post-menopausal discharge with some blood in it - be encouraging about you or them seeing a doctor about it. From what I've read, this doesn't only occur in older women either. There is plenty online about the occurrence of this in young women, so it might be your daughter or niece who needs to be informed about it.

Whatever your own circumstances, something brought you to this short book, and got you to this page. I am not a medical professional and whatever I've shared in these words is only my experience and brief memory of things that were explained to me. Do not take my words or experience as the basis of establishing your own medical requirements. Please - learn the signs, do some research, and spread the word.

Endometrial Cancer - Carcinoma of the Endometrium.

It's worth checking out, and keeping the signs in the back of your mind. It might come in handy in your own health. It might come in handy when a woman you care about talks to you and mentions one little thing that's happened to her that's out of the ordinary.

Whatever brought you here today, thank you for reading this.

Olivia Tusk